# The Seven-Day Gallbladder Diet Plan For Vegans

Jerry V. Hatcher

# Table of Contents


Introduction ..................................................... 1

Chapter 1: Wholesome Recipes for Gallbladder

Wellness for Vegans ........................................ 3

Chapter 2: Seven day meal plan .................................. 29

Conclusion ..................................................... 33

About the author .............................................. 35

My Little Request ............................................. 37

# Introduction

In the intricate symphony of human physiology, the gallbladder plays a vital role as a small yet indispensable instrument. Nestled beneath the liver, this pear-shaped organ undertakes the task of storing bile—nature's emulsifier—until it's summoned to aid in the digestion of fats. Just as a finely tuned instrument requires care to perform at its best, so does the gallbladder demand attention and mindful nourishment to maintain its health and functionality.

The Seven-Day Gallbladder Diet Plan For Vegans emerges as a guiding light for those seeking to cultivate balance and well-being within their digestive system while adhering to a vegan lifestyle. This dietary strategy emphasizes the consumption of plant-powered foods that are gentle on the gallbladder, reducing the risk of gallstones and promoting optimal digestion. Bursting with nutrient-rich whole grains, plant-based proteins, fresh fruits, and vegetables, this diet finds its strength in a harmonious blend of vegan ingredients that honor both taste and health.

Navigating the realms of plant-based gastronomy, this diet becomes an exploration of flavors, textures, and cruelty-free ingredients that not only invigorate the palate but also fortify the body. From the robust flavors of Quinoa and Vegetable Breakfast Bowl to the delicate balance of Chocolate Avocado Mousse, each dish showcases the potential for culinary excellence while nurturing the gallbladder's needs in a vegan context.

This plant-based gallbladder diet is more than just a collection of vegan recipes; it's an invitation to embark on a journey of self-care and mindful nourishment within the bounds of a vegan lifestyle. By choosing plant-powered, gallbladder-friendly ingredients, you empower yourself to embrace a compassionate lifestyle that fosters vitality and digestive wellness. Throughout this guide, you'll discover a diverse array of delectable vegan creations, from comforting soups to vibrant salads and enticing plant-based entrees, all thoughtfully designed to support your gallbladder's health.

Join us as we delve into a seven-day exploration of vegan flavors and nourishment, celebrating the gallbladder's unique role in our well-being. From tantalizing your taste buds to embracing the wisdom of holistic health within a vegan framework, The Seven-Day Gallbladder Diet Plan For Vegans invites you to experience the harmonious union of mindful eating and cruelty-free culinary delight. Let us embark on this vegan journey together, honoring our bodies and savoring each delicious plant-powered moment along the way.

# Chapter 1: Wholesome Recipes for Gallbladder Wellness for Vegans

1. Quinoa and Vegetable Breakfast Bowl

   - A hearty breakfast option with quinoa, sautéed spinach, cherry tomatoes, and avocado, providing a good mix of fiber and nutrients.

Ingredients:

- 1 cup quinoa, rinsed

- 2 cups water

- 2 cups fresh spinach, chopped

- 1 cup cherry tomatoes, halved

- 1 avocado, sliced

- Salt and pepper to taste

Instructions:

1. In a saucepan, combine quinoa and water. Bring to a boil, then reduce heat, cover, and simmer for 15-20 minutes or until quinoa is cooked and water is absorbed.

2. In a skillet, sauté spinach until wilted.

3. Assemble the bowl: place cooked quinoa in a bowl, top with sautéed spinach, cherry tomatoes, and sliced avocado.

4. Season with salt and pepper to taste.

2. Creamy Zucchini Soup

   - A smooth and comforting soup made with zucchini, potatoes, and a touch of nutritional yeast for a creamy texture.

Ingredients:

- 4 medium zucchinis, sliced

- 2 potatoes, peeled and diced

- 1 onion, chopped

- 4 cups vegetable broth

- 2 tbsp nutritional yeast

- Salt and pepper to taste

Instructions:

1. In a large pot, sauté onions until translucent.

2. Add zucchinis, potatoes, and vegetable broth. Bring to a boil, then simmer until vegetables are tender.

3. Use an immersion blender to puree the soup until smooth.

4. Stir in nutritional yeast and season with salt and pepper.


3. Chickpea and Spinach Salad

   - A protein-packed salad featuring chickpeas, fresh spinach, cherry tomatoes, cucumber, and a light lemon-tahini dressing.

Ingredients:

- 1 can (15 oz) chickpeas, drained and rinsed

- 4 cups fresh spinach

- 1 cup cherry tomatoes, halved

- 1 cucumber, sliced

- 2 tbsp tahini

- 1 tbsp lemon juice

- Salt and pepper to taste

Instructions:

1. In a large bowl, combine chickpeas, spinach, cherry tomatoes, and cucumber.

2. In a small bowl, whisk together tahini and lemon juice to create the dressing.

3. Pour the dressing over the salad and toss to coat.

4. Season with salt and pepper.


4. Millet-Stuffed Bell Peppers

  - Roasted bell peppers filled with a mixture of cooked millet, black beans, corn, and spices, creating a flavorful and satisfying dish.

Ingredients:

- 4 large bell peppers, halved and seeds removed

- 1 cup cooked millet

- 1 can (15 oz) black beans, drained and rinsed

- 1 cup corn kernels

- 1 tsp cumin

- 1 tsp chili powder

- Salt and pepper to taste

 Instructions:

1. Preheat the oven to 375°F (190°C).

2. In a bowl, mix together cooked millet, black beans, corn, cumin, chili powder, salt, and pepper.

3. Stuff each bell pepper half with the millet mixture.

4. Bake for 25-30 minutes or until peppers are tender.


5. Lemon-Dill Baked Tofu

   - Tofu marinated in a zesty lemon and dill mixture, then baked to perfection, providing a delicious and protein-rich main course.

Ingredients:

- 1 block extra-firm tofu, pressed and cubed

- 2 tbsp olive oil

- 2 tbsp lemon juice

- 1 tbsp soy sauce

- 1 tsp dried dill

- 1 tsp garlic powder

- Salt and pepper to taste


Instructions:

1. Preheat the oven to 375°F (190°C).

2. In a bowl, whisk together olive oil, lemon juice, soy sauce, dill, garlic powder, salt, and pepper.

3. Toss cubed tofu in the marinade until well-coated.

4. Place the tofu on a baking sheet and bake for 25-30 minutes or until golden and crispy.

6. Cauliflower Rice Stir-Fry

   - A low-carb alternative to traditional rice, stir-fried with colorful vegetables, tofu, and a ginger-soy sauce.

Ingredients:

- 1 medium-sized cauliflower, grated

- 2 cups mixed vegetables (bell peppers, broccoli, carrots)

- 1 block firm tofu, diced

- 3 tbsp soy sauce

- 1 tbsp sesame oil

- 1 tsp ginger, minced

- 2 cloves garlic, minced

Instructions:

1. In a large wok or skillet, sauté tofu until golden brown. Remove from the pan and set aside.

2. In the same pan, stir-fry mixed vegetables until tender-crisp.

3. Add grated cauliflower, soy sauce, sesame oil, ginger, and garlic. Cook for an additional 5-7 minutes.

4. Mix in the cooked tofu and serve.


7. Sweet Potato and Lentil Curry

   - A hearty curry made with sweet potatoes, lentils, and a blend of aromatic spices, served over brown rice.

Ingredients:

- 2 cups sweet potatoes, peeled and diced

- 1 cup red lentils, rinsed

- 1 onion, chopped

- 1 can (14 oz) coconut milk

- 2 tbsp curry powder

- 1 tsp turmeric

- Salt and pepper to taste

Instructions:

1. In a large pot, sauté onions until translucent.

2. Add sweet potatoes, lentils, coconut milk, curry powder, turmeric, salt, and pepper.

3. Bring to a boil, then reduce heat and simmer until sweet potatoes and lentils are cooked through.

8. Mushroom and Spinach Stuffed Portobello Caps

   - Large portobello mushrooms stuffed with a mixture of sautéed mushrooms, spinach, garlic, and breadcrumbs, baked until golden.

Ingredients:

- 4 large portobello mushrooms, stems removed

- 2 cups mushrooms, finely chopped

- 2 cups fresh spinach, chopped

- 2 cloves garlic, minced

- 1 tbsp olive oil

- Salt and pepper to taste

Instructions:

1. Preheat the oven to 375°F (190°C).

2. In a skillet, sauté chopped mushrooms, spinach, and garlic in olive oil until cooked down.

3. Stuff each portobello cap with the sautéed mixture.

4. Bake for 20-25 minutes or until mushrooms are tender.

9. Lemon Herb Quinoa Salad

   - A refreshing salad featuring cooked quinoa, fresh herbs, cherry tomatoes, cucumber, and a lemon vinaigrette.

Ingredients:

- 2 cups cooked quinoa

- 1 cup cherry tomatoes, halved

- 1/2 cup cucumber, diced

- 1/4 cup fresh parsley, chopped

- 2 tbsp olive oil

- 1 tbsp lemon juice

- Salt and pepper to taste

Instructions:

1. In a large bowl, combine cooked quinoa, cherry tomatoes, cucumber, and parsley.

2. In a small bowl, whisk together olive oil and lemon juice.

3. Pour the dressing over the salad and toss to combine.

4. Season with salt and pepper.

10. Baked Acorn Squash with Maple Glaze

   - Acorn squash halves baked with a drizzle of maple syrup, creating a sweet and savory side dish.

Ingredients:

- 2 acorn squashes, halved and seeds removed

- 2 tbsp maple syrup

- 2 tbsp olive oil

- 1 tsp cinnamon

- Pinch of nutmeg

- Salt to taste

Instructions:

1. Preheat the oven to 400°F (200°C).

2. In a bowl, mix together maple syrup, olive oil, cinnamon, nutmeg, and salt.

3. Brush the inside of each acorn squash half with the maple glaze.

4. Bake for 30-40 minutes or until the squash is tender.

11. Cucumber Avocado Gazpacho

   - A chilled soup made with cucumber, avocado, tomatoes, and a hint of jalapeño for a refreshing and hydrating option.

Ingredients:

- 2 cucumbers, peeled and chopped

- 2 avocados, peeled and pitted

- 3 tomatoes, chopped

- 1/2 red onion, finely diced

- 1 jalapeño, seeds removed and minced

- 2 cloves garlic, minced

- 1/4 cup fresh cilantro, chopped

- 3 cups vegetable broth

- 2 tbsp lime juice

- Salt and pepper to taste

 Instructions:

1. In a blender, combine cucumbers, avocados, tomatoes, red onion, jalapeño, garlic, cilantro, vegetable broth, and lime juice.

2. Blend until smooth.

3. Season with salt and pepper to taste.

4. Chill in the refrigerator for at least 2 hours before serving.


12. Roasted Brussels Sprouts with Balsamic Glaze

   - Brussels sprouts roasted to perfection and drizzled with a balsamic glaze for a flavorful and antioxidant-rich side.

Ingredients:

- 1 lb Brussels sprouts, trimmed and halved

- 2 tbsp olive oil

- 2 tbsp balsamic glaze

- Salt and pepper to taste

1. Preheat the oven to 400°F (200°C).

2. Toss Brussels sprouts in olive oil, salt, and pepper.

3. Roast for 20-25 minutes or until Brussels sprouts are caramelized.

4. Drizzle with balsamic glaze before serving.


13. Cilantro Lime Cauliflower Rice

   - A zesty and low-calorie alternative to traditional rice, seasoned with fresh cilantro and lime juice.

Ingredients:

- 1 medium-sized cauliflower, grated

- 1 tbsp coconut oil

- 2 tbsp fresh cilantro, chopped

- 1 lime, juiced

- Salt to taste

Instructions:

1. In a large skillet, heat coconut oil over medium heat.

2. Add grated cauliflower and cook for 5-7 minutes, stirring occasionally.

3. Stir in chopped cilantro and lime juice.

4. Season with salt to taste.


14. Pumpkin and Black Bean Chili

   - A hearty chili made with pumpkin, black beans, tomatoes, and chili spices, served over quinoa or rice.

Ingredients:

- 1 can (15 oz) black beans, drained and rinsed

- 1 can (15 oz) pumpkin puree

- 1 can (14 oz) diced tomatoes

- 1 onion, chopped

- 2 cloves garlic, minced

- 2 tsp chili powder

- 1 tsp cumin

- Salt and pepper to taste

 Instructions:

1. In a pot, sauté onions and garlic until softened.

2. Add black beans, pumpkin puree, diced tomatoes, chili powder, cumin, salt, and pepper.

3. Simmer for 15-20 minutes, stirring occasionally.

15. Green Goddess Kale Salad

   - A nutrient-packed salad featuring kale, avocado, pumpkin seeds, and a creamy green goddess dressing.

Ingredients:

- 6 cups kale, stems removed and chopped

- 1 avocado, sliced

- 1/4 cup pumpkin seeds

- 1/4 cup tahini

- 2 tbsp lemon juice

- 1 clove garlic, minced

- Salt and pepper to taste

Instructions:

1. In a large bowl, massage kale with avocado until it softens.

2. Add pumpkin seeds.

3. In a small bowl, whisk together tahini, lemon juice, garlic, salt, and pepper.

4. Drizzle the dressing over the salad and toss to coat.

16. Turmeric-Ginger Carrot Soup

   - A vibrant soup made with carrots, turmeric, ginger, and coconut milk, offering anti-inflammatory properties.

Ingredients:

- 4 cups carrots, peeled and chopped

- 1 onion, chopped

- 2 cloves garlic, minced

- 1 tbsp fresh ginger, grated

- 1 tsp ground turmeric

- 4 cups vegetable broth

- 1 can (14 oz) coconut milk

- Salt and pepper to taste

 Instructions:

1. In a large pot, sauté onions, garlic, and ginger until fragrant.

2. Add carrots, turmeric, vegetable broth, and coconut milk.

3. Bring to a boil, then reduce heat and simmer until carrots are tender.

4. Blend the soup until smooth using an immersion blender.

5. Season with salt and pepper.


17. Baked Eggplant with Tomato and Basil

   - Sliced eggplant baked with layers of tomato, basil, and a touch of nutritional yeast, creating a savory dish.

Ingredients:

- 2 medium-sized eggplants, sliced

- 2 cups cherry tomatoes, halved

- 1/4 cup fresh basil, chopped

- 2 cloves garlic, minced

- 3 tbsp olive oil

- Salt and pepper to taste

 Instructions:

1. Preheat the oven to 400°F (200°C).

2. Arrange eggplant slices on a baking sheet.

3. In a bowl, toss cherry tomatoes, basil, garlic, olive oil, salt, and pepper.

4. Spread the tomato mixture over the eggplant slices.

5. Bake for 20-25 minutes or until eggplant is tender.

18. Sesame-Ginger Broccoli Stir-Fry

   - Broccoli florets stir-fried with sesame oil, ginger, and soy sauce, providing a quick and flavorful side dish.

Ingredients:

- 4 cups broccoli florets

- 1 red bell pepper, sliced

- 1 cup snap peas, trimmed

- 2 tbsp soy sauce

- 1 tbsp sesame oil

- 1 tbsp fresh ginger, grated

- 2 cloves garlic, minced

 Instructions:

1. In a wok or large skillet, stir-fry broccoli, red bell pepper, and snap peas until crisp-tender.

2. In a small bowl, whisk together soy sauce, sesame oil, ginger, and garlic.

3. Pour the sauce over the vegetables and toss to coat.

4. Cook for an additional 2-3 minutes.


19. Mango-Avocado Salsa with Quinoa Chips

   - A refreshing salsa made with mango, avocado, red onion, and cilantro, served with homemade quinoa chips.

Ingredients:

- 2 ripe mangoes, diced

- 1 avocado, diced

- 1/4 cup red onion, finely chopped

- 1 jalapeño, seeds removed and minced

- 1/4 cup fresh cilantro, chopped

- Juice of 2 limes

- 1 cup cooked quinoa chips

Instructions:

1. In a bowl, combine diced mangoes, avocado, red onion, jalapeño, cilantro, and lime juice.

2. Mix gently.

3. Serve the salsa with quinoa chips.

20. Cauliflower and Chickpea Coconut Curry

   - A creamy coconut curry featuring cauliflower, chickpeas, and a blend of aromatic spices, served over basmati rice.

Ingredients:

- 1 head cauliflower, cut into florets

- 1 can (15 oz) chickpeas, drained and rinsed

- 1 onion, chopped

- 3 tbsp curry powder

- 1 can (14 oz) coconut milk

- 2 tbsp tomato paste

- Salt and pepper to taste

 Instructions:

1. In a large pot, sauté onions until translucent.

2. Add cauliflower, chickpeas, curry powder, coconut milk, tomato paste, salt, and pepper.

3. Simmer until cauliflower is tender.

4. Serve over basmati rice.

21. Baked Lemon-Pepper Asparagus

   - Asparagus spears seasoned with lemon zest, black pepper, and a touch of olive oil, baked until tender.

Ingredients:

- 1 bunch asparagus, trimmed

- 2 tbsp olive oil

- Zest of 1 lemon

- 1 tsp black pepper

- Salt to taste

 Instructions:

1. Preheat the oven to 400°F (200°C).

2. Toss asparagus in olive oil, lemon zest, black pepper, and salt.

3. Arrange on a baking sheet.

4. Bake for 12-15 minutes or until asparagus is tender-crisp.

22. Turmeric Roasted Cauliflower

 - Cauliflower florets tossed with turmeric, cumin, and coriander, then roasted to create a flavorful and colorful side dish.

Ingredients:

- 1 head cauliflower, cut into florets

- 3 tbsp olive oil

- 1 tsp ground turmeric

- 1 tsp ground cumin

- 1 tsp ground coriander

- Salt and pepper to taste

 Instructions:

1. Preheat the oven to 425°F (220°C).

2. In a bowl, toss cauliflower with olive oil, turmeric, cumin, coriander, salt, and pepper.

3. Spread on a baking sheet.

4. Roast for 20-25 minutes or until cauliflower is golden brown.

23. Spinach and Artichoke Stuffed Mushrooms

   - Mushrooms filled with a mixture of sautéed spinach, artichokes, garlic, and vegan cream cheese, baked until bubbly.

Ingredients:

- 16 large mushrooms, stems removed

- 2 cups fresh spinach, chopped

- 1 can (14 oz) artichoke hearts, drained and chopped

- 1/2 cup vegan cream cheese

- 2 cloves garlic, minced

- Salt and pepper to taste

 Instructions:

1. Preheat the oven to 375°F (190°C).

2. In a skillet, sauté spinach and garlic until wilted.

3. In a bowl, combine sautéed spinach, chopped artichoke hearts, vegan cream cheese, salt, and pepper.

4. Stuff each mushroom with the mixture.

5. Bake for 15-20 minutes or until mushrooms are tender.

24. Cabbage and Apple Slaw with Dijon Dressing

- A crunchy slaw made with shredded cabbage, sliced apples, and a tangy Dijon mustard dressing.

Ingredients:

- 1/2 head green cabbage, shredded

- 2 apples, julienned

- 1/4 cup red onion, thinly sliced

- 1/4 cup Dijon mustard

- 2 tbsp apple cider vinegar

- 2 tbsp maple syrup

- Salt and pepper to taste

Instructions:

1. In a large bowl, combine shredded cabbage, julienned apples, and sliced red onion.

2. In a small bowl, whisk together Dijon mustard, apple cider vinegar, maple syrup, salt, and pepper.

3. Pour the dressing over the slaw and toss to coat.

4. Chill before serving.

25. Chocolate Avocado Mousse

   - A rich and creamy dessert made with ripe avocados, cocoa powder, and a touch of sweetener, offering a guilt-free indulgence.

Ingredients:

- 2 ripe avocados

- 1/2 cup cocoa powder

- 1/4 cup maple syrup

- 1 tsp vanilla extract

- Pinch of salt

- Fresh berries for garnish (optional)

Instructions:

1. In a food processor, blend avocados until smooth.

2. Add cocoa powder, maple syrup, vanilla extract, and salt. Blend until creamy.

3. Spoon the mousse into serving bowls.

4. Chill in the refrigerator for at least 1 hour.

5. Garnish with fresh berries before serving.

Adjust portion sizes and ingredients based on individual dietary needs and preferences. Enjoy creating these delicious and gallbladder-friendly vegan recipes!

# Chapter 2: Seven day meal plan

Below is a suggested Seven-Day Gallbladder-Friendly Vegan Meal Plan using the twenty-five recipes:


Day 1:

Breakfast: Quinoa and Vegetable Breakfast Bowl

Lunch: Sweet Potato and Lentil Curry

Dinner: Lemon-Dill Baked Tofu with Roasted Brussels Sprouts

Snack: Lemon Herb Quinoa Salad


Day 2:

Breakfast: Cucumber Avocado Gazpacho

Lunch: Chickpea and Spinach Salad

Dinner: Pumpkin and Black Bean Chili with Cilantro Lime Cauliflower Rice

Snack: Sesame-Ginger Broccoli Stir-Fry

Day 3:

Breakfast: Millet-Stuffed Bell Peppers

Lunch: Turmeric-Ginger Carrot Soup with a side of Baked Lemon-Pepper Asparagus

Dinner: Mushroom and Spinach Stuffed Portobello Caps with Green Goddess Kale Salad

Snack: Mango-Avocado Salsa with Quinoa Chips


Day 4:

Breakfast: Creamy Zucchini Soup

Lunch: Lemon Herb Quinoa Salad

Dinner: Cauliflower and Chickpea Coconut Curry with Turmeric Roasted Cauliflower

Snack: Baked Acorn Squash with Maple Glaze


Day 5:

Breakfast: Chocolate Avocado Mousse

Lunch: Baked Eggplant with Tomato and Basil

Dinner: Cabbage and Apple Slaw with Dijon Dressing and Spinach and Artichoke Stuffed Mushrooms

Snack: Quinoa and Vegetable Breakfast Bowl


Day 6:

Breakfast: Sweet Potato and Lentil Curry

Lunch: Chickpea and Spinach Salad

Dinner: Pumpkin and Black Bean Chili with Cilantro Lime
Cauliflower Rice

Snack: Sesame-Ginger Broccoli Stir-Fry


Day 7:

Breakfast: Cucumber Avocado Gazpacho

Lunch: Turmeric-Ginger Carrot Soup with a side of
Baked Lemon-Pepper Asparagus

Dinner: Mushroom and Spinach Stuffed Portobello Caps
with Green Goddess Kale Salad

Snack: Mango-Avocado Salsa with Quinoa Chips


Feel free to adjust the portions based on your individual
needs, and don't forget to stay hydrated by drinking
plenty of water throughout the day. This meal plan aims
to provide a variety of flavors and nutrients while

adhering to gallbladder-friendly principles. This is just a sample, so remember that you can adjust these meals according to your preferences.

# Conclusion

As we conclude this journey through the pages of  The Seven-Day Gallbladder Diet Plan For Vegans  cookbook, let us pause to reflect on the profound connection between mindful nourishment and holistic well-being. In embracing this culinary adventure, you have not only discovered a plethora of delicious, plant-powered creations but also embarked on a path of self-care that extends far beyond the kitchen.

Remember, each meal you prepare is an act of love and nourishment for your body, a celebration of the intricate dance between flavors and health. By choosing the vibrancy of plant-based Ingredients, you have not only supported your gallbladder's health but also contributed to the well-being of our planet and all its inhabitants.

As you continue to savor the delightful tastes and textures presented in this cookbook, may you find joy in the kitchen, discovering the infinite possibilities of compassionate, gallbladder-friendly cooking. Cherish each moment spent creating these dishes, and relish in the knowledge that you are nurturing both your body and the world around you.

This is more than a cookbook; it is an invitation to cultivate a lifestyle filled with vitality, compassion, and balance. Celebrate the union of mindful eating and cruelty-free culinary delight, and may these recipes inspire you to embrace a life where each meal is an affirmation of your commitment to well-being.

So, dear reader, continue this journey with a heart full of love for yourself, for the planet, and for the countless delightful moments that mindful, plant-based cooking can bring. Here's to a future filled with vibrant health, boundless compassion, and the joy of savoring each delicious moment along the way. Bon appétit, and may your culinary adventures be ever nourishing and fulfilling.

# About the author

Jerry V. Hatcher is a culinary virtuoso and the creative
mind behind a collection of exquisite cookbooks that
transcend the ordinary. With a passion for gastronomy
and a flair for culinary artistry, Jerry has crafted a series
of cookbooks that take readers on a delectable journey
through the world of flavors.

Through his cookbooks, Jerry V. Hatcher combines the
finest ingredients with meticulous instructions, ensuring
every recipe is a delightful masterpiece waiting to be
savored. From tantalizing appetizers to mouthwatering
main courses and divine desserts, each page is a
celebration of culinary excellence.

With a keen eye for detail, Jerry's cookbooks go beyond
the recipes, providing valuable tips, techniques, and
personal insights that elevate the cooking experience to
new heights. Whether you're a seasoned chef or a
culinary enthusiast exploring the kitchen for the first
time, Jerry's books cater to all skill levels, fostering
confidence and creativity in every home cook.

Each recipe in Jerry V. Hatcher's cookbooks is a
reflection of his commitment to authenticity and a
passion for diverse cuisines. Drawing inspiration from
global flavors and local delicacies, Jerry's culinary

creations celebrate the richness of cultures and the joy of sharing food with loved ones. Indulge your passion for cooking and elevate your culinary skills with the culinary masterpieces crafted by Jerry V. Hatcher. Get ready to embark on a gastronomic adventure that will leave you hungry for more, one delicious recipe at a time.

# My Little Request

If you have gotten to this point, chances are high you have finished this book.

Thank You for Reading My Book!

I love hearing what you have to say.

I need your input to make the next version of this

book and my future books better.

Please take two minutes now to leave a helpful review on Amazon letting me know what you thought of the book

Thanks so much!

- Jerry V. Hatcher